I0440863

Playtime At The Dom Den; A Step-by-step Guide

ISBN-13: 978-1481824354
ISBN-10: 148182435X

Erotic BDSM Books - Your Erotic BDSM Book Publisher
EroticBDSMbooks.com

BDSM Books by Phil G Include:

*BDSM Master/slave Contract
*Mistress/slave BDSM Contract
*The Absolutely Essential Book of BDSM and S&M Rules
*Things To Do During 3 Hours of Sex; A Step-by-step Guide
*Playtime At The Dom Den; A Step-by-step Guide
*The Absolutely Essential Guide to Great BDSM and S&M Sex
*The Absolutely Essential Dominant/submissive Playtime Experience
*The Absolutely Essential BDSM Sexual Experience
*The Ultimate Collection of S&M and BDSM Rules For Female Submissives and Slaves
*Master and submissive or slave BDSM Contract
*The Funniest BDSM Personal Ads
*Have Awesome BDSM Sex
*Spanking Dictionary
*Spanking Contract
*BDSM Rules
*Bed Arrest, the Punishment for BDSM Enthusiasts

This book comes with two additional free bonus books (making it a $20.85 total value!) Your books are presented in this order:

Book 1

100 Great Lines To Put in Your Personal Ad

Introduction

The lines in this book can be combined with other lines you may think of to make your personal ad all it can be. Some lines in the book might need adapting to best suit you and/or your sex.

TAGLINES: Your short "tagline" is a headline that, perhaps along with your picture, can get readers to further explore your ad. Great taglines are like gold and people have paid hundreds of dollars for them! Now however many are on the Internet for you to see and use.

Remember, people love to laugh. A funny tagline is a big plus.

There is a great deal of material in this book to build quality taglines from. You may also want to take a bit of time and do a web search for "best personal ad taglines" for ideas. Chances are others (including those looking at your ad) haven't seen the tagline already, or have forgotten it if they did.

The Lines

A day not in love is a lost opportunity.

My friends know me as spontaneous, spritely, and upbeat.

I am searching for a beautiful person inside and out.

Are you looking for real love and someone special?

I enjoy thought provoking dialogue.

Together let's seek our destiny.

I hope only to fulfill your every desire. Is that too much to ask?

I love making people happy and to see them smile, even if at times it is at my own expense.

I feel the most pleasure when I know I am doing/enduring something to please another.

I'm looking to learn, not just to play....

I'd like to explore hidden fantasies with you.

I want to be taken to that special place and beyond.

I have the financial and emotional capacity to take care of myself.

Unlike perhaps others here I'm not misrepresenting myself. I know the importance of honesty.

I love sex. Rough sex, fun sex, emotional sex... I want you to respect me before and after but during is negotiable.

I want to explore my naughty side.

I'm looking for a friend, confidant and lover.

Like me I'd like you to be thoughtful, attractive, and looking to expand yourself as a person.

I have developed intricate pleasure techniques which can slowly arouse and pleasure beyond imagination.

I think I would describe myself, briefly, as quite a sociable person with a good sense of humor who doesn't take herself too seriously...having said that I believe I am also thoughtful and caring and someone who places great value on good friendships and relationships.

I am loyal, compassionate and respectful of people and animals. People describe me as easy going and good natured.

I have got great plans and goals in my life which I want to achieve.

I'm a contemporary yet spiritual soul in search of his charming, compassionate and caring companion to share this journey of life.

Are you looking for someone to grow with and push things further?

I have a wise mind and younger spirit.

I am an easy going, and loyal friend.

I'm looking forward to a fantastic voyage of a relationship.

I am attracted to someone who enjoys learning and growing.

Are you looking for fun, adventure and a challenge? If so I'm your girl.

I'm a passionate person with interests numerous and diverse.

I am trustworthy, affectionate, passionate, loving and non-judgmental. I am happy with myself and my accomplishments.

I want someone kind, loving, honest, communicative and self-aware. Your developed interest in education, hygiene, aesthetics, style and emotional literacy would make life easier for us. I'd like to find someone interested in building a relationship based on an accomplished life and a win/win attitude.

I am looking for someone who can work themselves deep inside my mind and make me fall to my knees.

Are you looking for someone to make you happy...someone that won't just have sex with you but will make love to you?

We all want to achieve heart pounding serenity.

I am looking for something more than just sex and games. Sure sex is a part of it but I also want someone that I can spend time with. I want the total package.

I want someone that I can go out with, talk with, laugh with, and fall in love with.

Outside of our playtime, I'd like to enjoy a harmony that can grow into a loving, trusting relationship. I enjoy the outdoors and staying healthy, going out on the town from time to time and hanging out at home.

My last relationship ended because we grew in different directions.

I am usually lucky and love life. I would like to find someone like that.

I'm a strong, seductive, passionate woman who is established and knows herself.

I'm well educated and well-travelled. I'm gainfully employed and very independent. I enjoy traveling, good food and wine, the theater and sports.

I'm searching for an open minded man with an adventurous soul and sensual heart. A journey in love is the destination. We still have plenty of time but none to waste! A beautiful world is waiting. Let's enjoy while we can!

I'll laugh at your corny jokes.

I'm a writer and voracious reader. I'm smart, and I like smart people.

Physical attraction leads to animal instincts.

I have a strong passion for the exploration and power of touch in all its forms.

I enjoy knowledge, I like to learn new and exciting things.

I am cosmopolitan and highly educated. I am a baby boomer, in good shape and would like an agemate and a partner who understands mutuality.

I am interested in developing a long term relationship.

I am interested in meeting someone who is honest, open and enjoys (his)her kink.

I have very many interests and I'm passionate about all of them! I love movies, literature, music, art, theatre, science… and lots of other things.

I am fun, open-minded, spontaneous and down for raunchy action.

The reason openness is important to me is that it shows that someone accepts themselves.

I'm lively and active and have a well developed sense of humor.

I hope to always be me and take advantage of any opportunities and chances whenever they're thrown at me.

I am totally devoted when in love.

I'm a laid-back, drama-free kind of person.

I want to be late to my own funeral.

Physical play is quite enjoyable but chemistry and a connection is more important.

I like to laugh, I like to have fun.

I believe that love is not what we see but what we do.

I won't ignore you or abandon you. I'm not looking for a secondary relationship.

I have a well developed and dominant sexual identity. I am seeking a man who is a smart, uninhibited, challenging partner.

I consider myself a natural leader, an innovator, a creator. I fight for the best and readily take the risks incumbent with leading a fulfilled, enriched life.

I am a strong, confident thinker, with a secure sense of himself (herself).

I consider myself to be a spontaneous, fun loving person. I work hard, play hard, and enjoy life. I'm a very affectionate and passionate. I like to hold hands and believe it or not cuddle. I believe in treating others the way I would like to be treated. I am looking for someone to grow with spiritually, mentally and physically. I want someone who is not afraid to love and be loved, someone who is affectionate, passionate and good kisser.

I will love you and take good care of you. I am someone who you can trust and believe in, someone who will always want to make you feel happy.

I'm neat and clean both internally and externally.

I want true love and real commitment.

I am looking for something more than just sex and games. There is a balance that is needed since none of us can live in a purely sexual world. Sure sex is an important part of it all but I also want someone that I can spend time with. I want the total package. I want someone I can go out with, talk with, laugh with, and fall in love with.

I want something that will naturally grow and evolve into its own very beautiful story.

I enjoy a great number of things and am very open to experimentation.

I'm interested in your fantasies.

I want to touch your body, your soul, your life.

I still believe that fairytales can come true, it can happen to us...

I live a healthy lifestyle. I am seeking the same.

I am brimming with sexual desire.

I will be looking forward to hear from you and Your wish will always be done...

I am looking for a partner - but I am happy to form a friendship.

Living on earth is expensive...but it does include free trips around the sun.

I eat healthy and workout regularly.

I am an educated, intelligent professional with eclectic tastes in most everything: art, music, food, people, entertainment and travel.

I'm looking for a non-smoker to share my life with in all ways, a friend and companion to travel with, commiserate over bad days and rejoice over good days; a lover and confidant.

Educated, professional and kinky.

I have class and style. I know the value of dressing to impress.

I would love to be able to say "I've finally found you."

I believe that we all have the ability to create or change anything.

I consider myself to be a sharp, crafty, inventive, fun, strong woman who enjoys life more when she's in a relationship.

I'm looking for a like minded man to chat, debate and play with.

I'm not a just fantasist wasting your time.

I am people biased not gender biased.

I am family-oriented and have family values.

I possess confidence but take pride in not being arrogant. I'm persistent but respectful. I have intelligence and charm.

I don't like negative people. We're here to live life not fear it.

I have learned in life that the smallest good deed is better than the grandest good intention.

I have high hopes for us.

I am a sharp, crafty, inventive, fun woman who doesn't hate men or hate anyone for that matter.

I enjoy life so much more when I'm in a relationship.

What you are like OUT of bed makes you more desirable for me to want you to take me there.

I like to please as much as be pleased.

I want to discover and explore my limits as well as push them further.

I like intellectual conversations.

My ambition is self-actualisation, to release the potential within.

I'm thoughtful, devoted, industrious, competitive, genuine and trustworthy.

I'm looking to learn and grow, not just to play....

End

Book #2 - The Absolutely Essential Guide to Erotic Breast Massage

Michelle Tallia

Copyright (C) 2013

The Absolutely Essential Guide to Erotic Breast Massage

The specialized breast massage discussed in this book can give a woman more pleasure than she can imagine. If her lover is unavailable to pleasure her this way, women can easily give themselves Extreme Pleasure Breast Massage, and the great news is it's something women can do to themselves for the rest of their lives.

There are a great many positions a woman's body can be in to receive this specialized and very sexually arousing breast massage. For this example though, let's have her sitting up and at least topless. Do note however that as she gets more and more aroused, she'd probably prefer to be naked so one or both of you can access her pubic area with fingers or toys while she's getting Extreme Pleasure Breast Massage.

For this position the massager sits behind her and up against her back. If it's okay with who is getting the massage, I suggest the massager be naked as many women will lose control at some point when getting Extreme Pleasure Breast Massage and be anxiously reaching behind their lower backs to play with the massager's privates. If a woman has never experienced this type of erotic massage before, she in particular may react with callous abandon.

Before placing yourselves in any of the massage positions, you'll need to have readily available a good supply of quality lotion, massage oil and/or hair conditioner. If using lotion, try to use some brand of non-desensitizing lotion. (Most lotions put desensitizers in them to dull the pain of dry skin and other irritations. These desensitizers can at least partially desensitize breasts thus cutting down on the breast's capacity to provide pleasure. Baby lotions at dollar stores sometimes are good ones to try but lotions tend to vary by brand. Another possibility to try is a thicker hair conditioner.) Cold lotion, massage oil or hair conditioner on breasts can provide an unwelcome jolt so if warming is necessary, warm the lotion/oil up ahead of time. You can also rub blobs of it in your hands to warm it up. Always have an ample amount of this massage oil or lotion nearby as well as well as small towels to wipe the oil/lotion off of your hands and her breasts after the massage is over.

Put a sizeable glob of massage oil/lotion on each of your hands, rubbing it all over your hands to spread it out, as well as warm it if it's not yet warm. Then put your well lubricated hands on her breasts, but not yet on her nipples and areolas! That is because those provide the most pleasure and thus the best is saved for last!

It is so important that the massager make sure to keep his/her massaging hands very well lubricated. When the oil or lotion is breaking down, the massager will feel stickiness developing. The rule of thumb is that you can't lubricate your hands and her breasts too much! Do note, it can cause irritation to the skin if it's not lubricated enough.

Also the massager needs to make sure his/her nails and skin of their hands are smooth. Trim and file your fingernails and that kind of thing, to as short and smooth as possible. Otherwise she (the person receiving the massage) might feel them as they rub against her sensitive skin. She can even get hurt by them because as she is in the thongs of ecstasy, she might not realize that they are hurting her, so make sure to watch out for her and take care of this situation.

Typically the massage will provide three levels of pleasure:

(a) Massaging the fleshy part of her breast (but not massaging her areolas and nipples) should give her pronounced and very welcome pleasure; (of course the faster her breasts are massaged, the more pleasure she'll get.)

(b) Including her areolas in the massaging will increase her pleasure a lot.

(c) But massaging her nipples and areolas at the same time will really get her going.

The following (and not in order of importance) are suggestions to optimize the breast massage.

* Start from the bottom of her breasts (where the breasts meet her torso) and work your way slowly higher up to just below her areolas. You can move your hands at varying speeds but typically the faster you massage the more pleasure she'll get.

* Simultaneously circle her boobs with each hand. Start out by using limited pressure on the breasts while utilizing only one finger, then gradually work your way up to utilizing all your fingers. Go clockwise then, counterclockwise (or vice-versa.) Remember, leave her nipples and areolas alone as much as possible until she's practically (or literally) begging for you to massage them. Sure you will "bump" into them from

time to time as you massage around them. Those bumps will give her a delicious taste of what's to come.

* At its base, wrap each hand around a single breast then run your well lubricated hands around and along that breast in a steady spiraling motion up the breasts in the direction of her nipples, until you reach the edge of her areolas. Of course you can go in the opposite direction also (starting from just below her areolas and working your way down to where her boobs meets her torso.)

* Place one hand on the base of one breast; the back of the hand should be facing her head. Put your other hand on the base of her other breast, the back of it should be facing her legs. Slide your well lubricated hands from left to right and then vice-versa, across and along both breasts.

* At its base, take each breast in a well lubricated hand and with increasing speed pull up from the base of her breast to the nipple until your fingers reach the edge of the areolas (or if you're already playing with her areolas and/or nipples, go all the way to her nipples.) Then do the opposite and slide your hands back down from the top of her breasts to the breast's base (where you started from.) Repeat this procedure many, many times.

* Tease her by sliding only your well lubricated fingertips over her breasts, wiggling your fingers.

* Instead of the above, perhaps for a minute or more, you'd like to start the festivities by teasing her breasts by only briefly touching them here and there using only the tips of your fingers.

* Concentrate your efforts on only one well lubricated breast; wrap both hands around it, kneading it, pulling it and twisting it.

As previously discussed, it's strongly suggested that you take your time before playing with her areolas and then nipples. This is because she will still get a good deal of pleasure from having the 'areola and nipple-less' massage. I for one require that she even beg you to play with her nipples--because as we know this is where the breasts offer the most pleasure. I would suggest waiting until she is already well stimulated. You may stroke her anticipation by whispering in her ear that you're about to play with her nipples, then suddenly do it. She may scream with delight as an orgasm overcomes her.

Playing with her nipples is typically the high point of her massage. She'll likely be getting the most pleasure now. (Again, the faster your well-lubricated fingers move around her nipples, the more pleasure she's likely to get.)

Okay massagers you now have a choice, you can immediately start massaging her nipples fast and hard, driving her crazy, or start massaging them slowly, then progressively massaging them faster and faster until she screams in ecstasy. If you're going to massage them fast immediately, as is the first option, many women will start their orgasm then (if they haven't already.)

Don't forget you can have her use a vibrator on herself as you massage her and thus it's suggested you keep a vibrator within arm's reach. Believe me she'll find it if it's there.

As noted previously, because so often the woman you're massaging will get so aroused from all this that with both hands she'll instinctively reach around her lower back to play with the massager's pubic area. She then will not have a free hand to use the vibrator on herself. Of course both your hands are busy giving her Extreme Pleasure Breast Massage. A way to counter this is to secure a vibrator with white medical tape (the type used to hold gauge and cotton to cuts etc.) over her most sexually sensitive pubic area. (Perhaps it would be helpful if she keeps her panties on for extra support.) If you do this, more women will orgasm while you are giving her this massage.

Remember guys her nipples can get tender after orgasm and need to be left alone for a bit of time. Also don't over massage her nipples and areolas or they can get raw.

As is obvious, ladies, you can give yourself Extreme Pleasure Breast Massage in the privacy of your bedroom.

After the massage, ladies your breasts tend to become firmer for a while and often they'll feel quite good for hours.

The following is another way of giving this massage, (told from the perspective of the kinky dominant massager.) Warning it is kinky!

We will go to the bed (if we're not already there.) I will set the bed up so I am sitting with my back against the headboard of the bed and you are

15

laying in front of me face-down on cushions with your head positioned so you can easily suck on my penis and play with my scrotum using your tied-together hands.

Also I'll put a roughly 3' x 3' sheet of plastic under your upper body to keep the massage lotion or oil from going on the bed covers. (More on this massage very soon!)

Perhaps I will also tie your bound hands to the headboard. If I do that though I will make sure there is enough slack in the rope for your hands to still move freely around my penis and scrotum while you suck. If your hands are tied to the headboard, I will be sitting on the rope as my butt will be in-between your bound hands and the headboard which your hands are tied to.

Your breasts will now be positioned, thanks to these cushions, literally just above the ground. As you suck on my penis, I will generously lubricate (and keep lubricated,) your breasts with some brand of preferably non-desensitizing lotion, massage oil or conditiner. I will warm the lotion/oil up ahead of time or rub it in my hands to warm it up, if warming is necessary. I will then massage your breasts. (Many lotions put desensitizers in them to dull the pain of dry skin. These can at least partially desensitize breasts thus cutting down on the breast's capacity to provide pleasure.) I will continue for a long time to massage your lubricated breasts as you suck on my penis. (Remember to always keep the massager's hands well lubricated!)

Using a yardstick type implement, I can reach across your back and spank you as you suck on my penis. Obviously one should make sure the woman can handle being spanked while sucking. Most can depending on the intensity of the spanking and how hard she's already orgasming.

End

This book is sold and/or distributed with the understanding that the publisher and author is not engaged in rendering legal or other professional services. **This book and its subject matter are for entertainment purposes only.** In this publication there may be inadvertent inaccuracies including technical inaccuracies, typographical inaccuracies and other possible inaccuracies. **The writer and publisher of this publication expressly disclaim all liability for the use or interpretation by anybody of information contained in this publication.** The author, publisher and distributors of this publication hereby disclaim any and all liability for any loss or damage caused by errors or omissions resulted from negligence, accident, or any other causes. If legal advice or other expert assistance is required, the services of a competent professional person in a consultation capacity should be sought. Products, services and websites' content vary with time. Please verify any published information.

Book #3 - Special Things To Do During 3 Hours of Sex; A Step-by-step Guide

Copyright (C) 2013

Please note that the following sexual experience has kinky overtones to it. If you find any of that disconcerting, please use alternative aspects of this sex scene. This is written from a male dominant perspective.

.

Playtime At The Dom Den; A Step-by-step Guide

I am a sexually dominant, heterosexual male. I need my lady love to be able to orgasm-on-demand, or agree to be trained for it. Typically she's trained to have extremely long orgasms versus several comparatively shorter ones. This is part of where my sexual dominance comes in. My lover will need to start her orgasm quickly, and continue it for as long as I am sexually stimulating her by using my hands or other parts of my body. Fortunately the human female body is built to have long, frequent and powerful orgasms, though so comparatively few women get to enjoy their incredible built-in capacity for pleasure. The truth is that orgasm-on-demand is a remarkably easy thing for women to do once properly trained.

Most men concentrate on a woman's body to stimulate her sexually, (which in and of itself is not a bad idea) but in so many cases that's not enough. I have found that most men do not adequately sexually stimulate their women's minds.

There is a natural tendency by women to be the more submissive sex during sexual activity, and that would certainly be required for the 3 hour playtime we're discussing. (Please note that if this tendency toward submissive behavior is not true in your case then this type of orgasm on demand training likely won't work too well with you.)

In her now sexually aroused state, it's normal for her subconscious mind to be more susceptible to suggestions regarding sex. People like me take it a step further and require her to do more than that during her sexual submission, specifically she will be required to orgasm long and hard, no ifs, ands or butts. Thus it is no longer her decision on how hard and long to orgasm but her lover's and I for one will require her to orgasm relentlessly.

Another way to look at it is that after being trained for orgasm on demand, the woman no longer is the one making the decision as to when she is going to have her orgasms and/or how intense the orgasm will be. She has yielded that responsibility to her lover and her mind fully accepts his/her authority in the matter.

Let's remember, a woman's subconscious mind doesn't usually care who tells it to begin orgasming, it can be her own mind giving the order or it can be her lover's. As a woman you just have to be in the right frame of mind to let it happen.

For 3 hours of sex it is very helpful if the man lasts a long time and/or is capable of getting hard frequently and with minimal downtime.

I last an extremely long time, usually for at least the whole 3 hours. I also have a thick penis which of course is a help.

Incidentally if someone is looking for an easy to find penis desensitizer cream, over the counter hemorrhoid cream under the tip of the penis can work well. I would urge the man to test it out on himself before being with a woman as if too much is used he might not even feel the stimulation enough to get hard! The man needs to know just what the right amount to use is and chances are it's a small amount.

I wanted to note that the dominant sexual position discussed in this book works best when the woman is no more than somewhat overweight.

Here are specifics of what we'd do in our 3 (or more) hour playtime.

1. When you enter my (our) place, you will take off your shoes and go kneel on the thick padding next to my bed (or other agreed upon spot like a chair or couch). Unless told otherwise, your eyes will be looking at where my midsection would be when I sit down in front of you. You will wait for me there (unless of course I'm already there.)

2. I will come over and sit in front of you (assuming I'm not already there.) I may or may not have clothes on. You'll then put your hands on my upper legs, massaging my legs with anticipation. Keep your hands high up on my legs, massaging my legs but you may not touch my penis until allowed to.

3. I will kiss you, touch you, play with you, talk to you and undress you as you kneel in front of me. At some point I may tell you to stand up and take the rest of your clothes off.

4. You will partially or fully undress me when I tell you to. When you pull my pants and underwear down, you know what will pop out!

5. I will then let you suck on my penis. You will first likely have to beg for it though. Also, remember to always play with my testicles while you suck…always!

Rule: Never let any of my penis' ooze go to waste. You know good it tastes! Beg me to let you check for ooze often! Keep sucking my ooze down until I tell you to stop.

6. Soon I will reach down and play with your exposed, vulnerable breasts as you suck on my penis.

7. At some point I may tell you to stop sucking my penis. If so I will then tie your hands securely together.

8. I may tell you to suck on my penis again or we will go straight to the following:

I will sit further back on the bed (or couch/chair) and you will lay stomach down across my lap. I will give you a nice sensual spanking, playing with your body as I do.

I will then tell you to get up and we will go to the bed (if we're not already there.) I will set the bed up so I am sitting with my back against the headboard of the bed and you are laying in front of me face-down on cushions with your head positioned so you can easily suck on my penis and play with my scrotum using your tied-together hands. If I do that though I will make sure there is enough slack in the rope for your hands to still move freely around my penis and scrotum while you suck. If your hands are tied to the middle of the headboard in this manner, I will be sitting on the rope as my butt will be in-between your bound hands and the headboard that your hands are tied to.

9. I'll also put a roughly 4' x 3' (though it can be larger) sheet of strong plastic under your upper body to keep the massage lotion or oil from going on the bed covers. (More on this massage very soon!)

Your breasts will now be positioned, thanks to cushions, so the bottom tips (which will likely be the nipples) of the breasts are just above the bed. As you are lying down and sucking on my penis, I will **generously** lubricate (and keep lubricated,) your breasts with some brand of preferably non-desensitizing lotion or massage oil. The longer the lotion can stay viscous, the better. If warming is necessary (which it most likely will be,) I will warm the lotion/oil up ahead of time or rub it in my hands to warm it up. I will then massage your breasts as you suck on my penis and play with my testicles.

I will continue for a long time to massage your lubricated breasts as you suck on my penis. (This is known as "Extreme Pleasure Breast Massage".) **Remember massagers, <u>always</u> keep you're your hands well lubricated!**

Massager and massagee will quickly notice that the nipples respond with the most pleasure from this type of massage. The massager will find that massaging his lady's breast's large fleshy area first for a while will be quite pleasurable to his slave but it is still not near as pleasurable as briskly massaging her nipples with a circular twisting motion that lets the fingers slide firmly over the nipple, not actually twisting it.

I will first make my lady beg to have her nipples massaged using this Extreme Pleasure Breast Massage technique. My lady has no more than 30 seconds to start her orgasm when I first start giving her Extreme Pleasure Breast Massage. Once I start massaging her nipples, she will have to orgasm a lot harder or risk being punished.

Using a yardstick type implement, I can also reach across your back and spank your bottom as you suck. Obviously one should make sure the woman can handle being spanked while sucking. Most can depending on the intensity of the spanking and how hard she's already orgasming.

Optional: After doing this massage for some time, you may wish for the lovely lady to be turned over on her back, her hands still tied to the bed. The man can then eat her. The lady should plan on providing her man with a lot of pussy juice. Should she not provide you with enough pussy juice, feel free to turn her over so her bottom is facing up, and give her a good spanking. Then try eating her again. (Before playing it is important that the lady keep her pussy clean and fresh.) After you've had your fill of her pussy juice, both of you can go back to the original position mentioned in this section or move on to #10.

10. At some point, I may also tie each foot to its corresponding corner of the bed. Instead I may tie your feet securely together and then tie them to the middle of the bed frame at the foot of the bed. Don't worry guys, the placement of a woman's vagina on her body while she's laying on her stomach is such that you still most likely will have easy access even with her legs closed. (However this could be a problem depending on how overweight she and/or he is.)

11. At some point I will order you to stop sucking by saying "head up". I may then get up and give you another spanking as you lay tied down, just for good measure. If you've been a good girl and are getting a lot of pleasure from all this, and if you beg for it, I will put a special vibrator (or two) inside and/or on you and set it up so it stays in place. (Tight underwear and white first aid fabric tape often work best where there are pubic hairs in the area.) I will then return to my original position on the bed and you will continue sucking me and I will also continue giving you Extreme Pleasure Breast Massage (which I promise you'll enjoy immensely!) I will continue to periodically spank you with a yardstick type implement as described earlier.

12. After a while, I will tell you to stop sucking. I'll then clean the lotion off your breasts with a small towel(s) and remove the small plastic sheet that caught lotion that came off your breasts and my hands. I'll also remove the cushions from under you that kept your breasts literally an inch above the bed. You are now comfortably laying face down on the bed but now without the cushions and plastic under you. You still however are tied down to the bed as you lie on your stomach. (You may wish to put a clean towel under her breasts if they are still a bit oily from the massage.) I will remove any vibrators on and/or in you, as well as whatever was holding them in place. You will be completely naked, tied down, vulnerable and ready to be taken.

13. I will come back in front of you and order you to suck on my penis again. After it is hard, I will dry it off (it must be completely dry for the condom to stay on) and put a condom on it. I will then lay on top of you, stomach down, and enter you with my thick penis.

14. As I take you, you will orgasm for as long as I order you to and orgasm as hard as I order you to. You are <u>required</u>, as part of the orgasm on demand training, to start orgasming within 5 seconds of me entering you. Believe me, it is much easier than it may sound. You will need to ask for permission to start orgasming though! As long as you start asking for permission within 5 seconds of me entering you, you are doing fine. Of course you will need permission to stop your orgasm also! There is the possibility that at some point I will order you to stop your orgasm during our lengthy playtime (or obviously you may have to do that due to unexpected events like the kids coming home early.) If you can however,

you are welcome to keep orgasming, even though direct sexual stimulation has temporarily stopped. Once direct sexual stimulation of your breasts and your vagina restarts, you'll of course have to re-start your orgasm once again (assuming it had stopped,) and within 5 seconds as always. (Many of the ladies I have trained will continue orgasming for minutes after physical sexual stimulation has stopped.)

15. As I take you, you will orgasm for as long as I order you to and orgasm as hard as I order you to. Believe me young lady, I require long, hard orgasms from you.

16. As you know I am taking you while both of us are on our stomachs. My stomach of course is on your back. This is far and away the main position I will take you in for the entire time I take you. I may also take you doggie style depending on how overweight she is. There will however not be an emphasis on multiple sex positions during our playtime.

RULE: while I'm playing with you, if you are lying on your stomach and if I ever say "elbows" you are to raise your chest enough so that the tips of your lovely breasts are just above the bed, thus making it easier for me to play with your breasts by sliding one or more of my hands under your chest as I am taking you.

(I think you'll find that my stomach on your back position to be a very good one. Depending on how heavy and/or tall the guy is, you won't have any trouble breathing as my weight is well distributed over your bone-protected pelvis. You won't have to deal with my breathing on your face or you being pounded against the headboard like in the missionary position. Also I can hold you tightly as I take you and easily talk to you as my mouth can be right by your ear.

17. At some point I will slide one or both of my arms under your underarm(s) and put my hands on or around your hands. I can now securely hold you down with my hands. You can now reach my hands (as they are on your wrist, forearms or hands) and kiss them should that be our desire.

18. Sometimes while I am taking you like this, I will spank you. This is accomplished best by me holding myself up with one hand/arm while I am in you and then spanking you with a paddle or the like with the other hand.

19. Often I will hold you down while I take you. I will order you to struggle FROM THE WAIST UP to get free as I am holding you down and taking you at the same time. We will do this one or more times during our long playtime.

20. Sometimes I will take you faster than other times. You will get even more pleasure from this as most any woman would.

21. Sometimes I will thrust into you as deep and hard as I can. You will get even more pleasure from this as most any woman would.

22. This is an excellent sex position for a lady to be taken anally. Perhaps she should have her anus lubed in the beginning when she is originally laid in place incase her man decides to take her anally.

RULE: Remember, the man must always wear a condom when taking her anally and he **can not** re-enter her vagina unless his pubic area has been thoroughly cleaned. A bladder infection is just one of the problems she can have if one doesn't abide by this essential safety tip.

Remember, if something is hurting young lady, you need to tell your man immediately so he can stop.

Well so there are the sexy details of how to play for 3 (or more) hours! Have fun!

The End

www.ingramcontent.com/pod-product-compliance
Lightning Source LLC
Chambersburg PA
CBHW071352310526
45790CB00018B/1421